A GUIDE TO CALMNESS WHEN YOU CAN'T THINK STRAIGHT

STOP THAT PANIC ATTACK RIGHT NOW

Ideas from hospice nurses, physical therapists, counselors, and teachers.

Exercises that work for anxiety sufferers of any age... from 3 to 103.

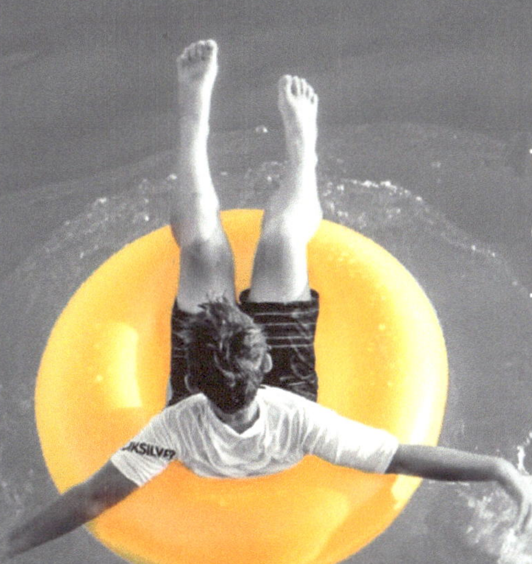

COMPILED BY: PHYLLIS DILLARD

Copyright 2018
by Phyllis Dillard

Stop That Panic Attack Right Now
ISBN-13: 978-1719250597
ISBN-10: 719250596

Printed in the USA

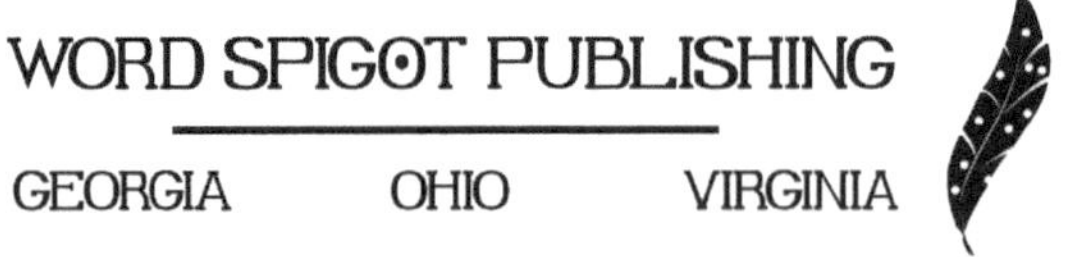

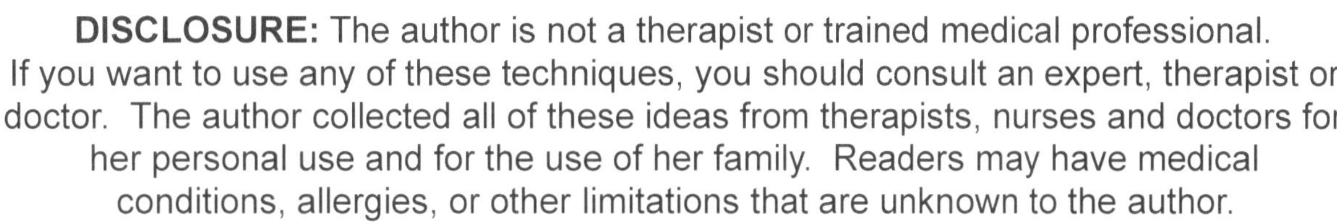

DISCLOSURE: The author is not a therapist or trained medical professional. If you want to use any of these techniques, you should consult an expert, therapist or doctor. The author collected all of these ideas from therapists, nurses and doctors for her personal use and for the use of her family. Readers may have medical conditions, allergies, or other limitations that are unknown to the author.

Introduction

Living with anxiety is never easy, but you are in good company. Like you, millions of people fight anxiety every day and they are all looking for relief. **Children** experience panic, **college age students** suffer with anxiety attacks, and **senior citizens** find themselves in the clutches of heart-racing fear in the middle of the night.

This book is a guide for people of any age when panic strikes. It will get you through to the other side. By the time you work through the techniques in this book, which will take 20 or 30 minutes, you will feel much better and will be able to return to what you *want* to be doing right now — sleeping, working, driving, relaxing, and enjoying your day. **You may not need to work through the whole book to experience a calmer mindset. Many times, just one exercise will work.**

Be Prepared

There are many books that define and describe panic attacks in great detail. This book does not try to repeat that work. Instead, it assumes you know that you are in a stage of life that produces panic attacks. This book simply guides you through a series of exercises that are designed to bring calm.

Health care workers can share this book with their patients as part of their treatment plan. When an anxiety sufferer is in the midst of an anxiety attack, it can be hard for them to recall the techniques their health care providers have advised them to try. Flipping through the pages of this book will give them a reminder.

Prepare now, while you are calm, by doing three things: read this book, gather supplies, and master "deep breathing."

Be Prepared
Read this book

Practice the exercises in this book when you are calm, so that when you are in the midst of a panic attack, you won't have to read the instructions. Instead, you can just be reminded of the calming techniques by glancing at the **bold print** and the illustrations. **When you are having a panic attack, start at the bright red page that is titled "Start Here."** Feel free to skip to the exercises that help you the most and do them in any order that works for you.

If you are an adult, you may feel a little silly doing some of these exercises, but going through the motions will activate a certain region of your brain that will calm your anxiety. You can imagine that you are entertaining a student or a grandchild, if that makes you feel less silly!

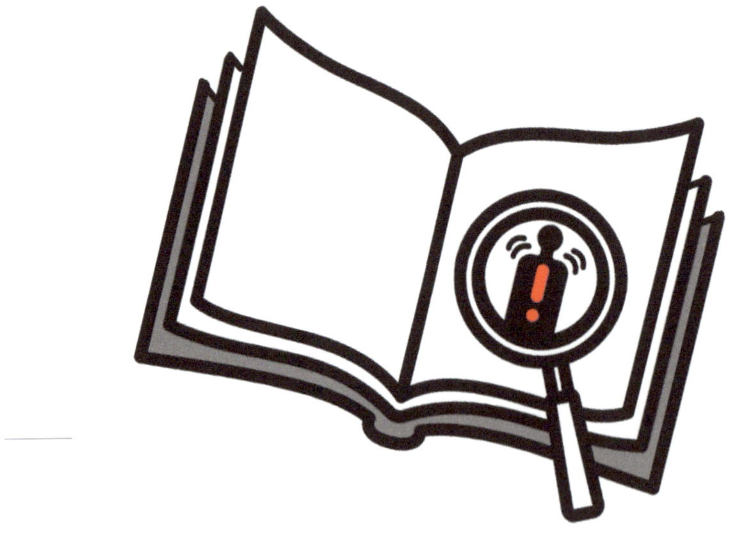

Be Prepared
Gather supplies

Have these items easily accessible in your kitchen and beside your bed, beside your favorite chair, in your desk drawer, in your bathroom, in your car, or wherever you most often have panic attacks.

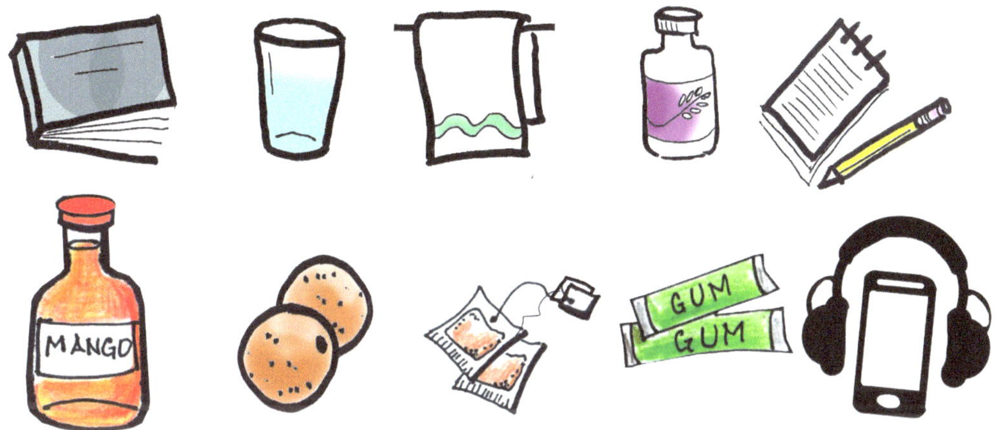

The Calming 10

This book.

A drink.

A washcloth.

Essential oils.

A pad of paper and pencil.

Mango juice.

Oranges.

Tea.

Peppermint gum.

Some mellow music.

Be Prepared
Learn Deep Breathing - Exercise 1

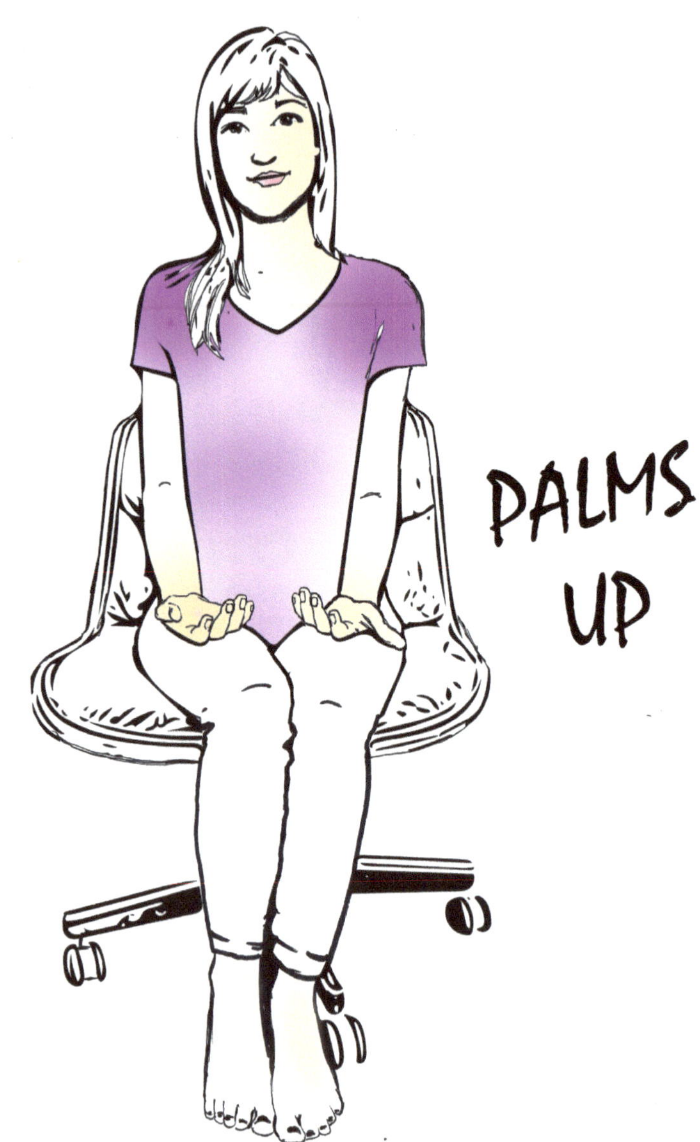

Sit up, tall and comfortable, with your palms up.

Keep your shoulders relaxed.

Your body follows your mind and your mind follows your breath.

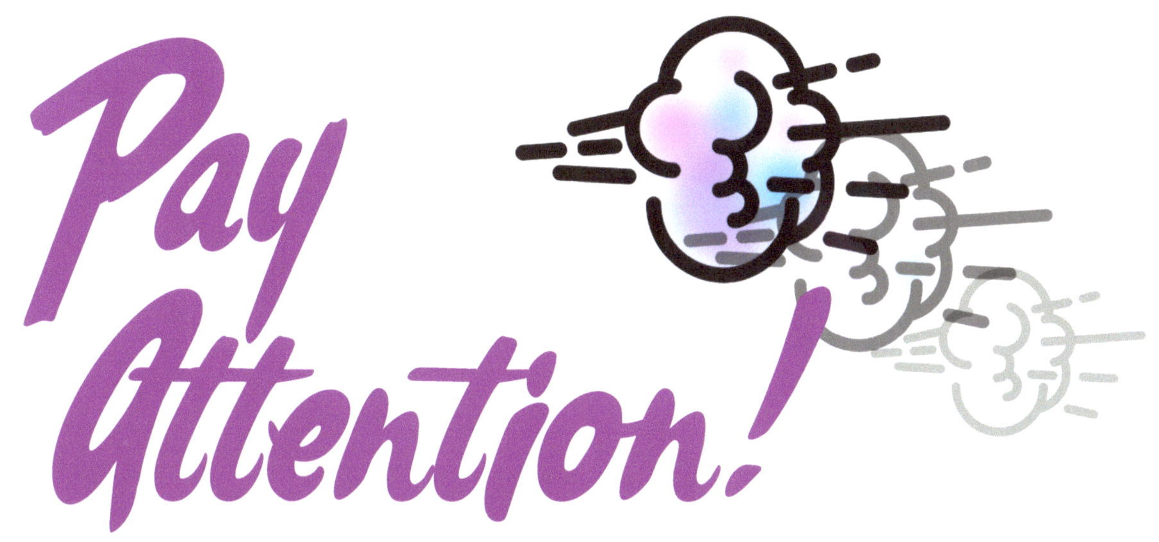

This exercise helps you recognize the difference between your normal breathing pattern and deep diaphragmatic breathing.

Notice your normal breathing pattern.
Close your eyes and pay attention to how you breathe normally. Where does your breath start - in your chest or your abdomen? Do your ribs move in and out? Are your muscles tight or loose? Do your breathe through your mouth or nose?

There is no right or wrong way to breathe. The point is to just be aware of your normal breathing pattern. **Deep breathing will feel different from your normal breathing.**

Be Prepared
Learn Deep Breathing - Exercise 2

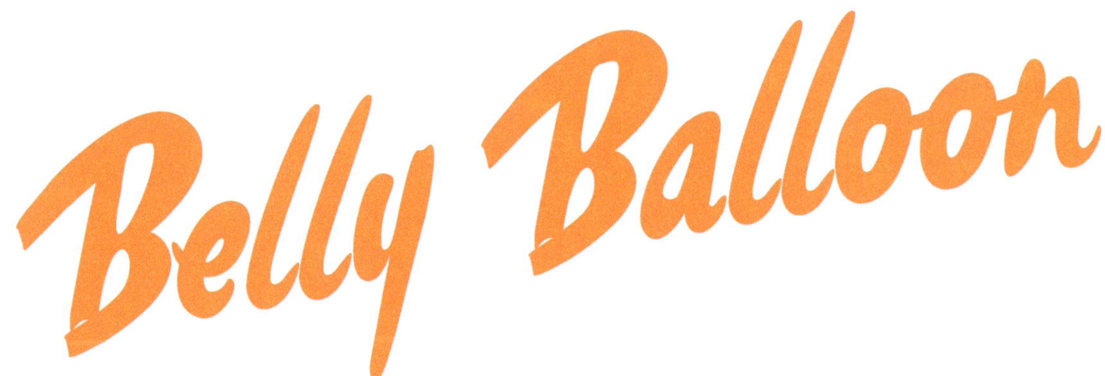

This exercise helps you correctly pace deep abdominal breathing.

Imagine there is a balloon of your favorite color on your belly. Put your hands on your belly and **inhale through your nose while you count, 1… 2… 3… 4,** and blow up that colorful, imaginary balloon on your belly.

Pause.

Exhale, through your nose or mouth, all the air in your belly balloon while you, **count 1… 2… 3… 4,** and squeeze your belly button all the way back to your spine.

Dizzy? Make sure that you are breathing into your belly.

Repeat 5 times.

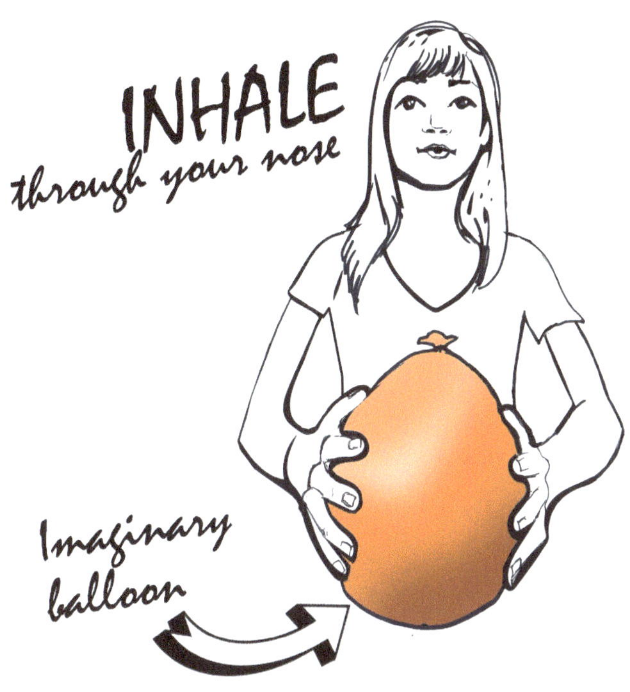

PAUSE

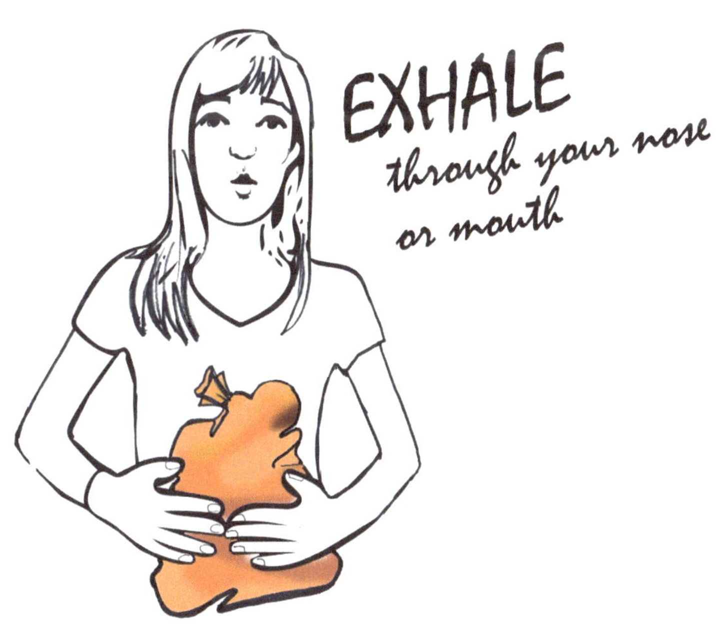

Deep belly breathing signals the nervous system to relax, lowering stress and regulating the heart rate and blood pressure.

Be Prepared
Learn Deep Breathing - Exercise 3

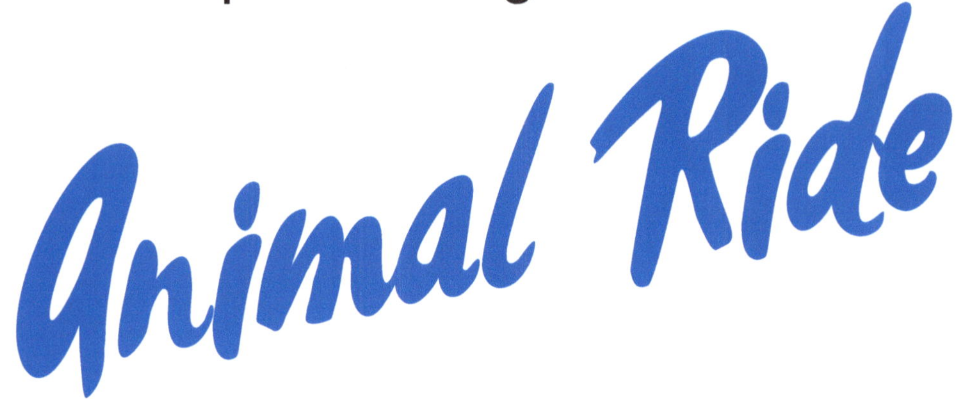

This exercise helps you to isolate the muscles that are activated when doing deep abdominal breathing correctly.

Lay on your back and place a stuffed animal or small pillow on your belly. As you count to four, inhale deeply through your nose, 1… 2… 3… 4, filling your belly with air and watching the object on your belly rise up.

Pause.

Exhale slowly as you count, 1… 2… 3… 4, watching the object on your belly come down.

Take your time between inhaling and exhaling. Try not to rush your breathing. **Dizzy?** Make sure that you are breathing into your belly.

Repeat 5 times.

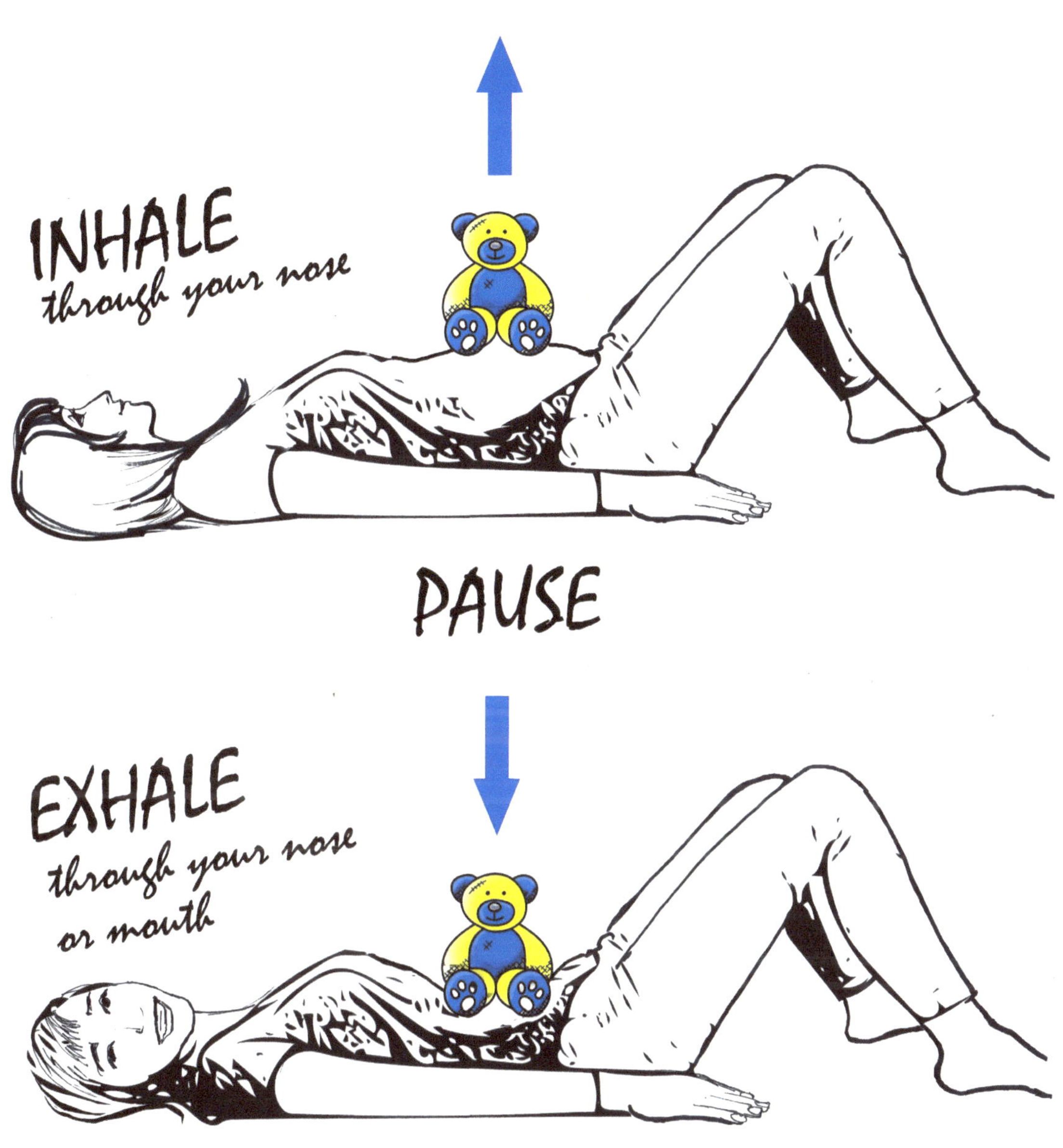

When you concentrate intently on the moment instead of your mind's worries, you chase away anxiety.

Start Here

to stop a panic attack.

First, calm your body.

Second, calm your brain.

**You may feel like you are having a hard time breathing.
You can change that!**

In the next few pages you will use the deep belly breathing
techniques you have practiced, to **control your breathing**.

Sit tall with your palms up.
Feel your belly expand with each inhalation.
Keep your shoulders relaxed.

Make a note of what time it is — you will be calmer in 20 minutes!

Calm your Body
Control your Breathing - Exercise 1

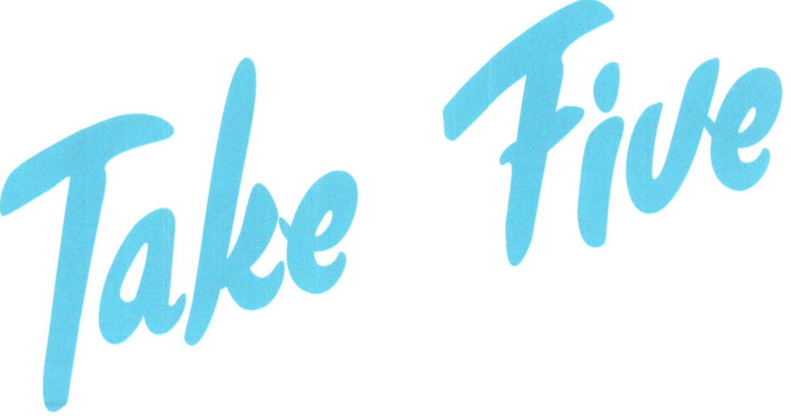

Stretch your fingers on one hand out like a star. Use the pointer finger of your other hand like a pencil and imagine tracing around the outline of your hand and fingers while breathing slowly and steadily. **Breathe in through your nose, then out through your mouth or nose.** Make sure you feel your belly, not your chest, expanding with each inhalation.

Follow the path shown in this illustration or use your finger to trace the illustration. Use the belly breathing technique and count, 1… 2… 3… 4, each time you inhale and exhale. If you are out in public, you can imagine you are tracing your hand while breathing deeply. Imaginary exercises can be just as calming as actually doing them!

Dizzy? Make sure that you are breathing into your belly.

Repeat 5 times.

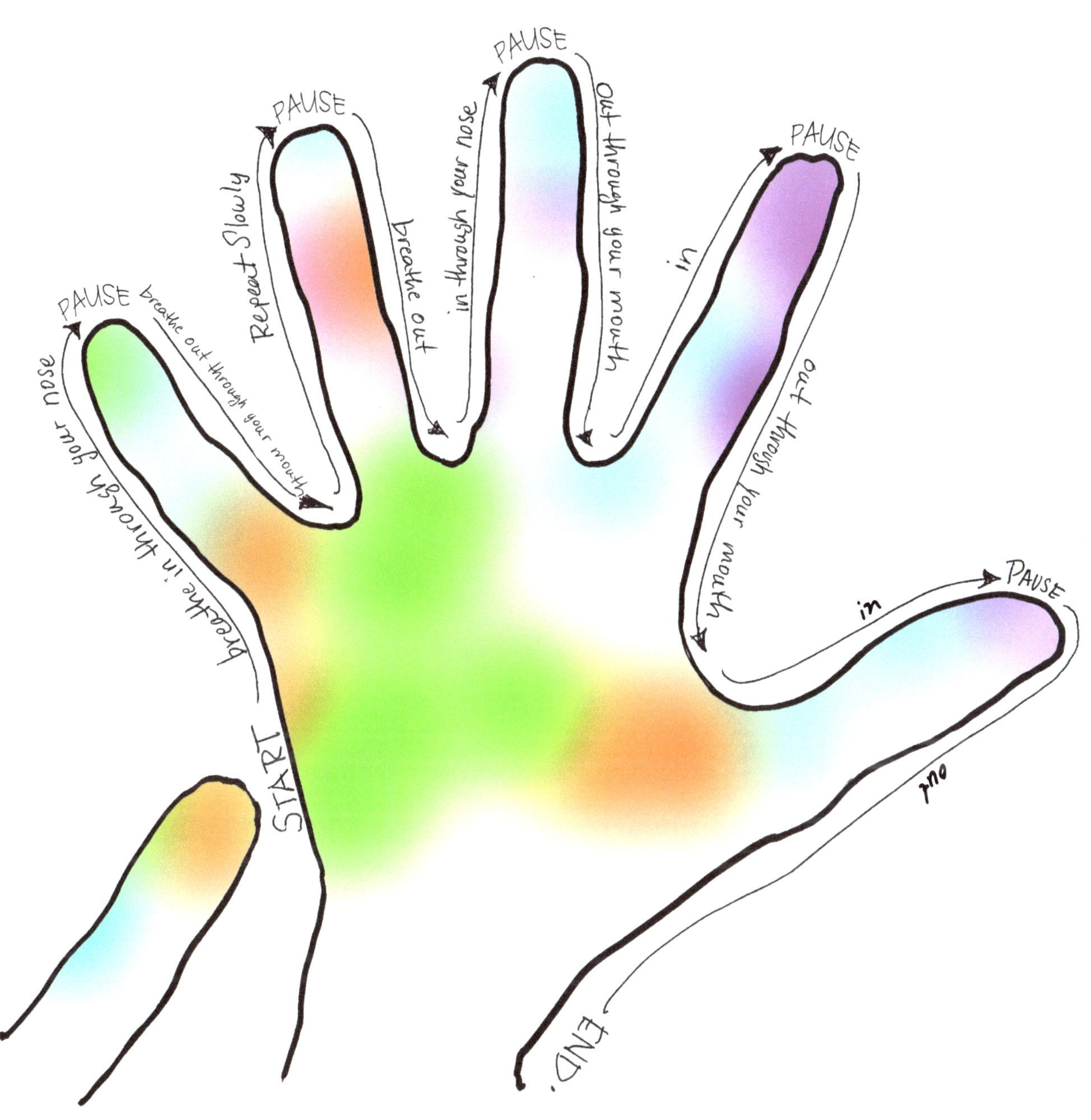

Use your pointer finger to trace your other hand.

Feel your belly expand.

Calm your Body
Control your Breathing - Exercise 2

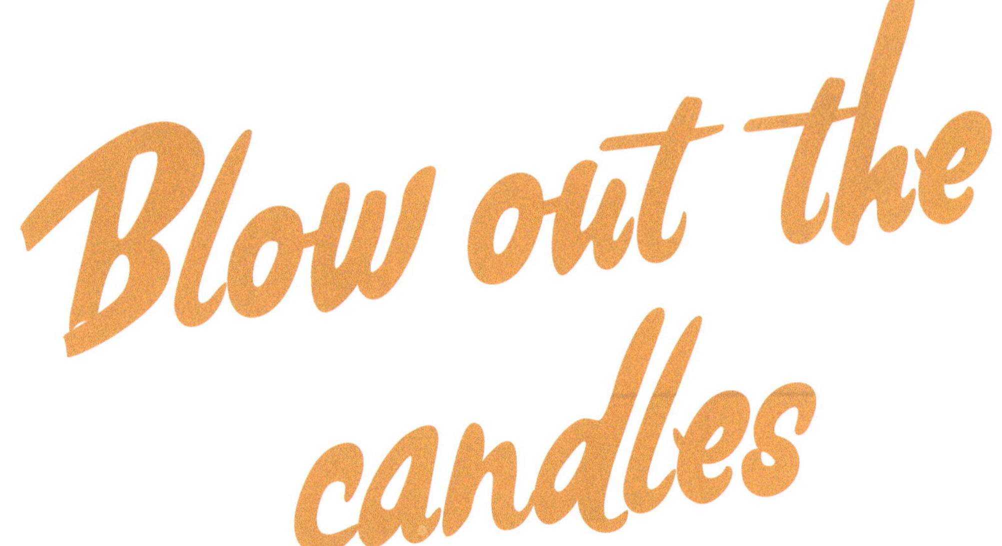

Stretch your fingers out like candles on a cake and slowly blow each "candle" out, tucking each finger into the palm after you blow. Use the belly breathing technique and count, 1… 2… 3… 4, each time you inhale and exhale as you blow out the imaginary candles.

This method of breathing will ensure that you are not hyper-ventilating (a common sensation of those with anxiety). It will help you regain the CO_2 balance in your body and alleviate many of the worst anxiety symptoms.

Dizzy? Make sure that you are breathing into your belly.

Repeat 5 times.

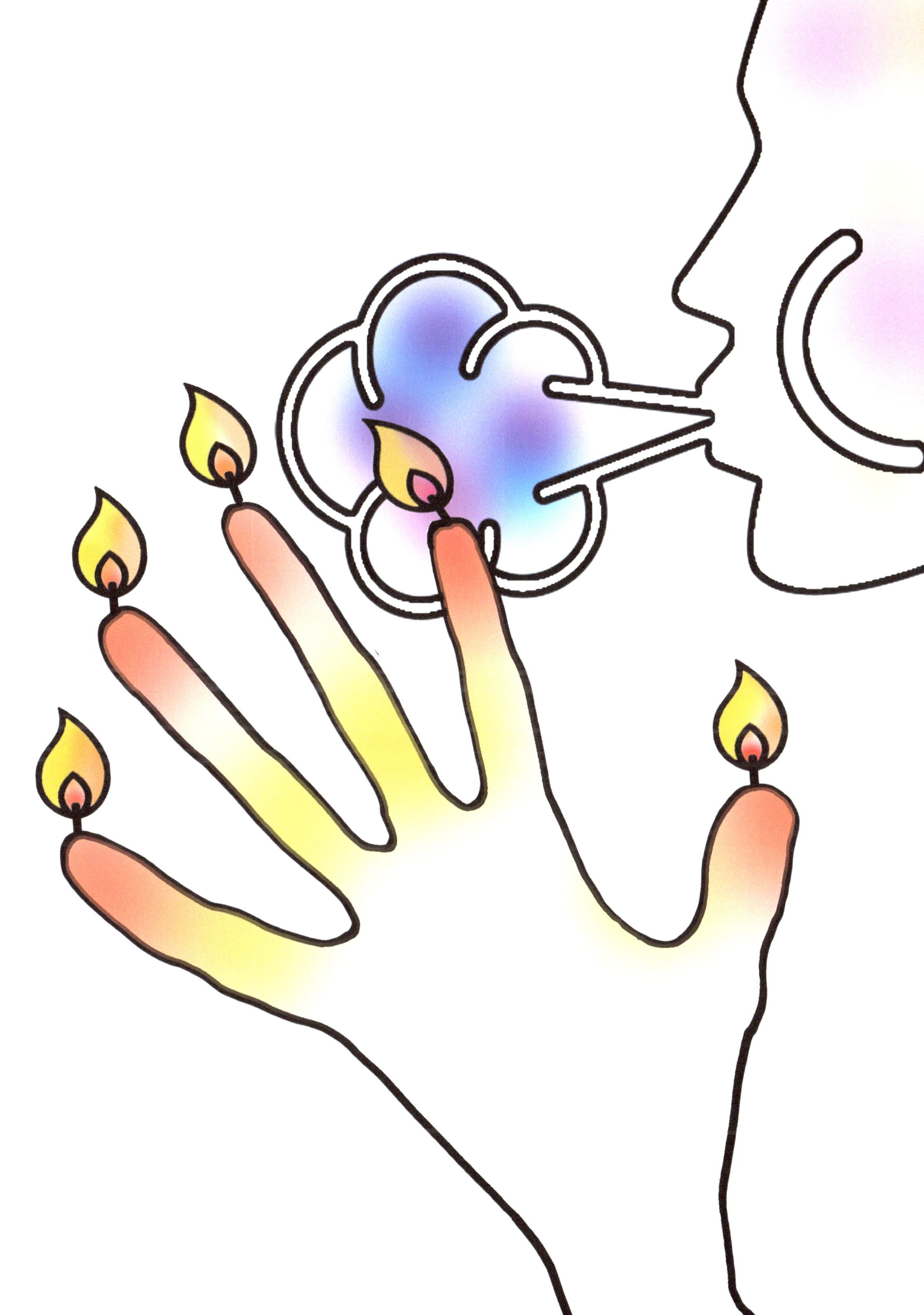

Calm your Body
Tense and Release

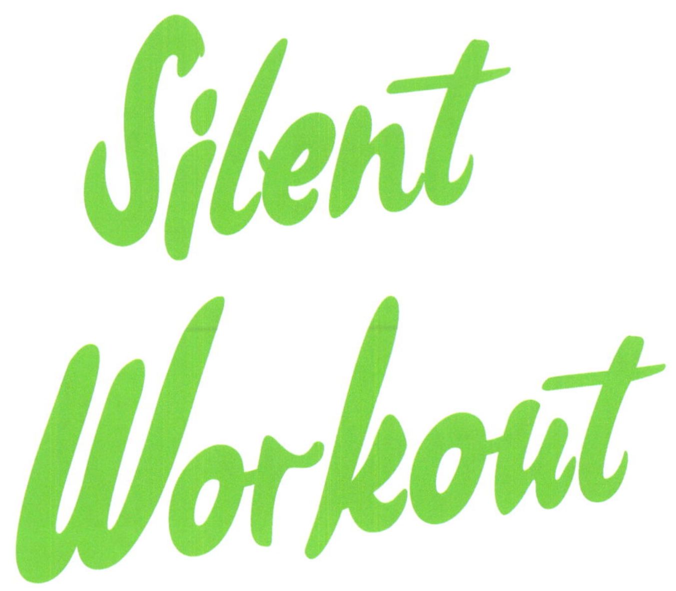

Exercise is the perfect antidote for panic. If you are able to do it, take a walk. Notice all the sights and sounds. Breathe in the fresh smell of grass, listen to the birds or to the sounds of your city.

However, there are many reasons that you may not be able to go out and walk around the block. When anxiety hits at bedtime, at work, at school, or anywhere else that you can't get active, you need to re-set your body and brain in a subdued way.

**Relax one muscle group at a time by tensing
and releasing them**.

Inhale deeply as you make your
legs straight and stiff.
Count to 4.
Exhale and relax your legs.

Inhale deeply as you squeeze your
hands into fists.
Count to 4.
Exhale and relax your hands.

Inhale deeply as you scrunch up
the muscles in your **face**.
Count to 4.
Exhale and relax your face.

Inhale deeply while your tense up
all your muscles.
Count to 4.
Relax and let your limbs go limp.

Repeat several times.
Notice how relaxed your body feels!

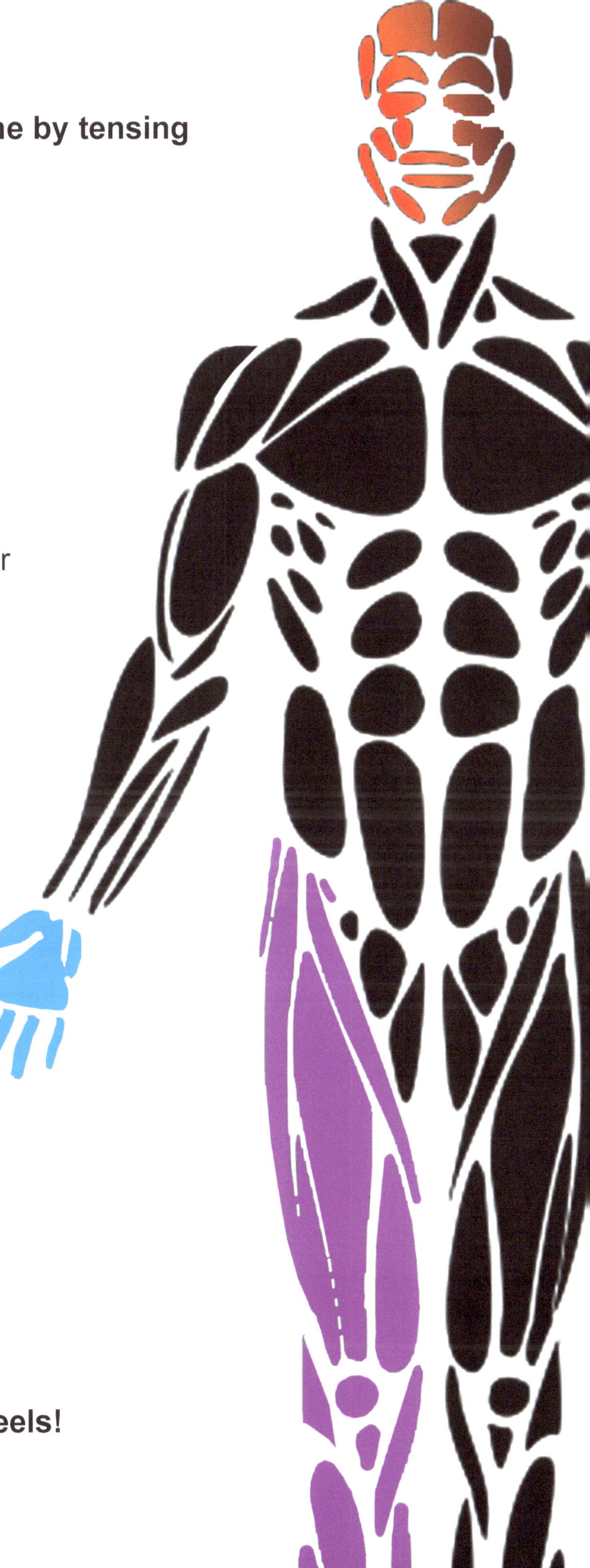

Transition Exercise
Thoughts

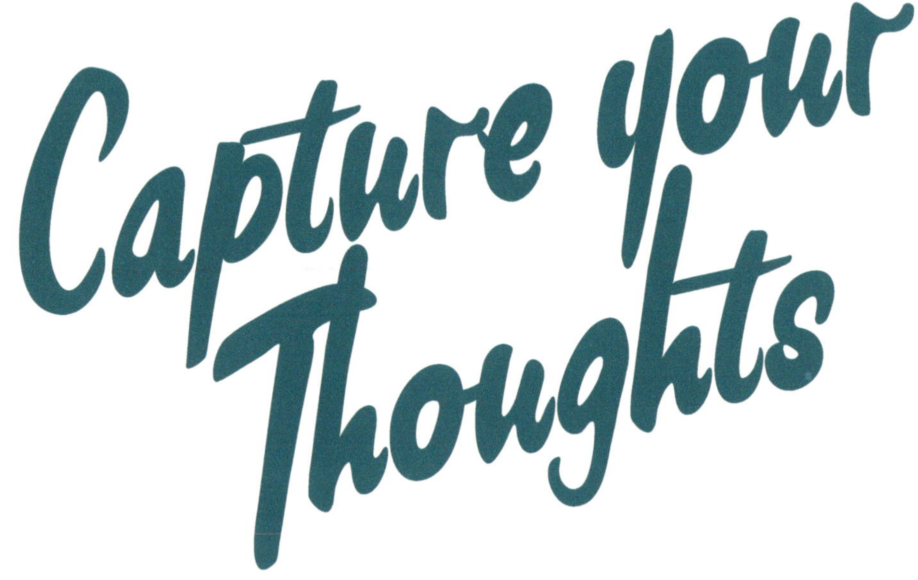

Now we will transition from calming your body to calming your mind. To start … **sing, sing a song.**

When asking friends and family how they cope with fearful, stressful events, they often mention activities that involve past **memorization or singing**.

One person says, "I sing a song I learned as a child, 'Perfect Peace,' whenever I have to go down to the scary cellar!"

Another friend reports, "I repeat the 23rd Psalm in my head when I need to calm down."

Make a list of your favorite scriptures, songs or poems.

You may still rememeber the Preamble to the Constitution. I am sure you remember childhood songs and your all-time favorite popular hits from your high school years.

Repeating words from memory (even silently to yourself) will engage your brain for a few minutes in this calming practice. Here's an example list:

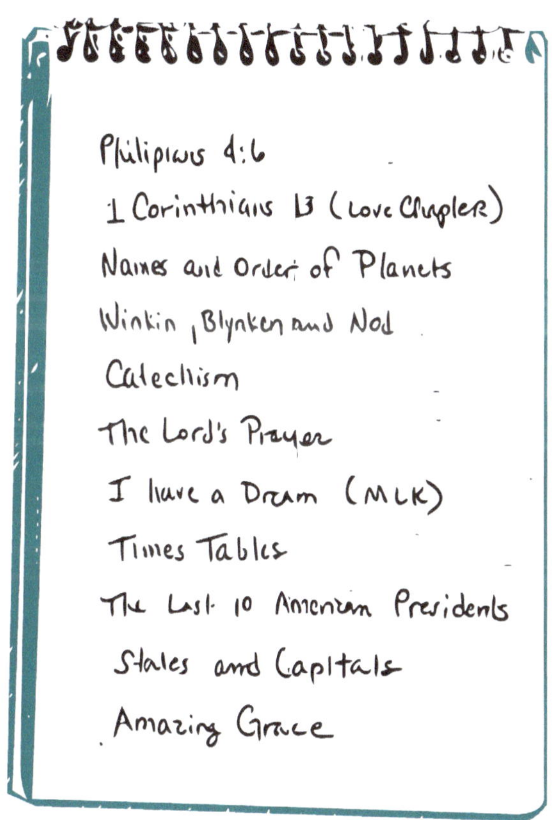

Meditation and Prayer:

If you are a person of faith, remember that prayer is a powerful tool to bring peace and calm!

Calm your Brain

The next few pages will guide you through **grounding exercises**. Your nervous system has a multitude of sensors, with one sensor dedicated to every sense and brain function. Your anxiety sensor is demanding attention right now! Grounding exercises calm you by attending to the other sensors and letting the anxiety sensor rest. You can do grounding exercises for these senses: taste, touch, smell, sight, and hearing. Next, you can add some brain games and mental exercises to activate sensors involved with memory.

Grounding Exercise
Sense of Taste

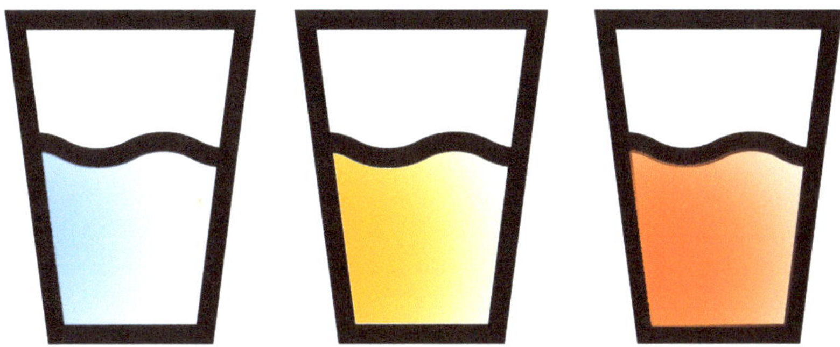

Get a healthy drink. Water is always a good choice, but mango juice (or a mango popsicle) is one of the best juices to kill stress because its full of B-complex vitamins, selenium, zinc, and potassium, all of which are proven anxiety killers.

Some anxiety sufferers claim that a cup of **hot tea** is their cure. You can sip your way to calmness and relaxation with peppermint, chamomile, lemon balm, passion flower, or lavender tea. (Check with your doctor - some teas can interact with medications.)

As you sip your drink, notice how it tastes and feels. Is it sweet? Tangy? Fruity? Cold? Hot? Is it soothing to your throat? Enjoy every sip!

One more taste trick: Peppermint chewing gum will cool your tounge and settle your nervous stomach.

Grounding Exercise
Touch

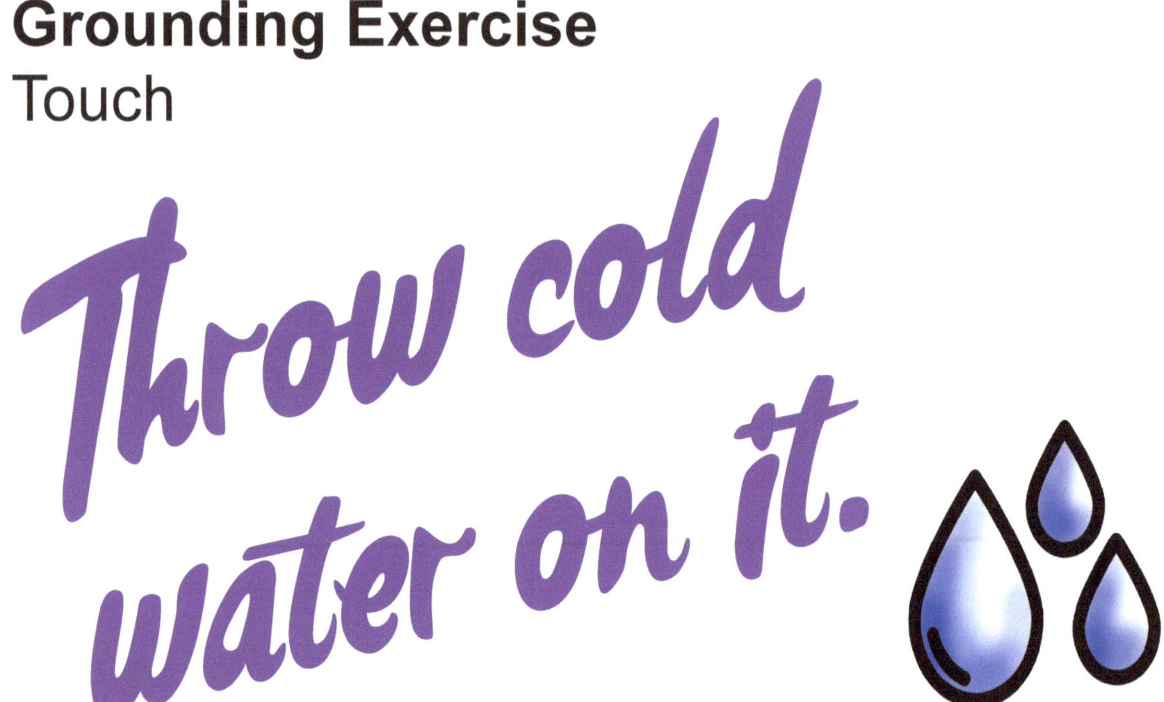

Get a cold washcloth.

Put a cold wash cloth behind your ears and on your wrists. The essential oil, lavender, has calming properties, so put a drop of it on your washcloth for some aromatherapy. Notice the texture of the washcloth and the refreshing feeling of the cold water. Splashing cold water on your skin can also change your physiology and mood. This is because wet and cold both cause your surface vessels to tighten, making blood move from your body surface to your core. This conserves body heat and floods the brain and vital organs with fresh oxygen-rich blood.

It is also calming to stroke a soft blanket or silky pillowcase. Babies are experts at calming themselves in this way!

Grounding Exercise
Smell

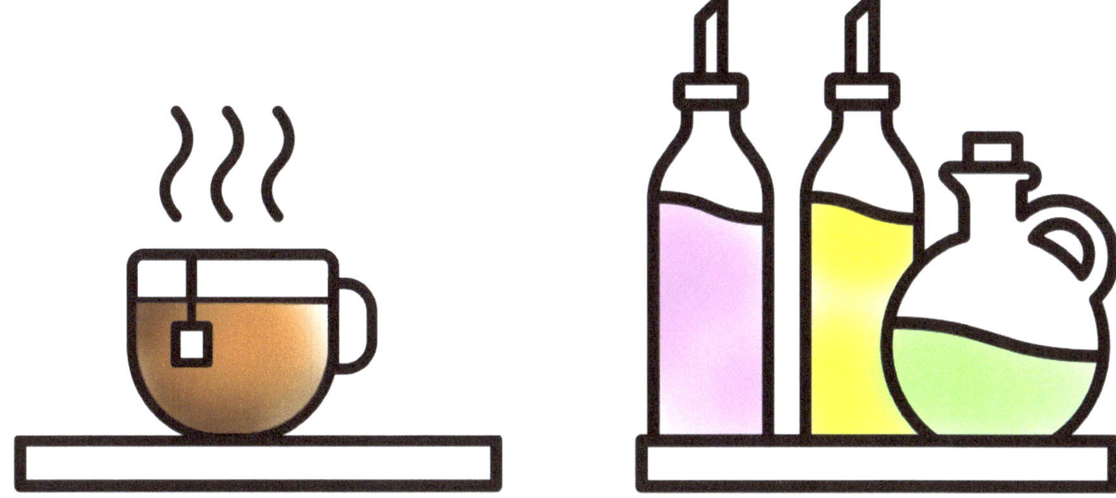

Notice what you can smell right now.

Do you smell dinner cooking? Rain on the way? Inhale deeply and notice the aromas that surround you. If the smells aren't that pleasing, you should make a change!

It is widely reported that the scent of oranges has a calming effect on many people. Try smelling some **freshly sliced oranges** to see if it helps you. Other calming scents are lemon, lavender, peppermint, rose oil, frankincense, and chamomile. These are available in teas and **essential oils,** which can be mixed into hand lotions or diffused into the room with a diffuser.

(Again, check with your doctor for possible drug interactions.)

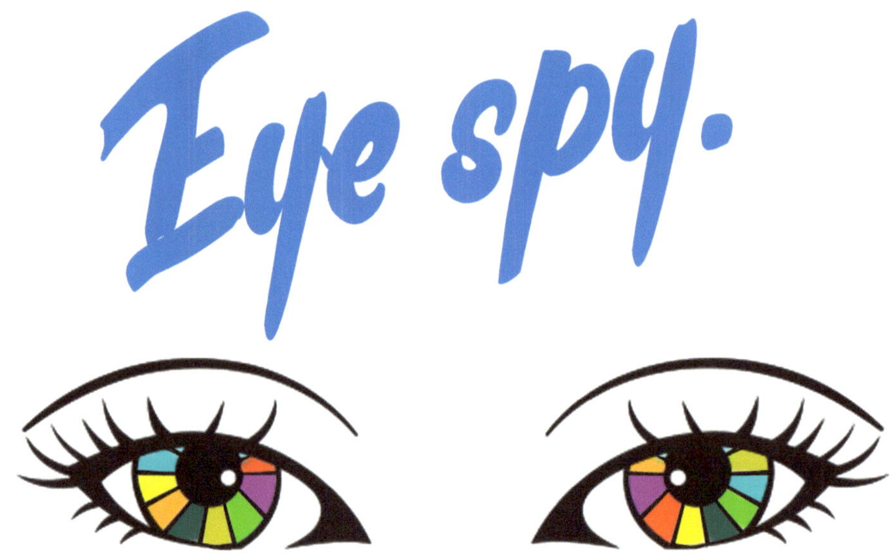

Look around you.

Find something **blue** within your sight.

Find something

brown.

Find something

green.

Find something

red.

Grounding Exercise
Sight

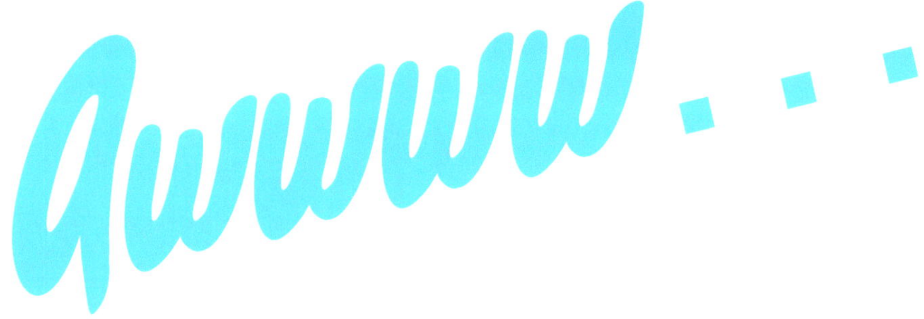

There is scientific evidence that viewing certain images can decrease stress and make you happier. Your vision tells you very quickly if the environment is safe, causing feel-good emotional responses, or if risky, causing anger or fear. A large part of your brain is required in processing what you see.

That is why looking at cute animals and babies makes people happy and less anxious. If you can't hug a real baby or puppy, close your eyes and remember a time that you did hold a fuzzy puppy or a warm baby. How did they smell? Were they wiggly or sleepy or soft? If you go online and look at funny baby animal videos and pictures, you will get a lasting positive mindset from this!

Imagine how this puppy's ears would feel to you.
What about that baby's fuzzy head?

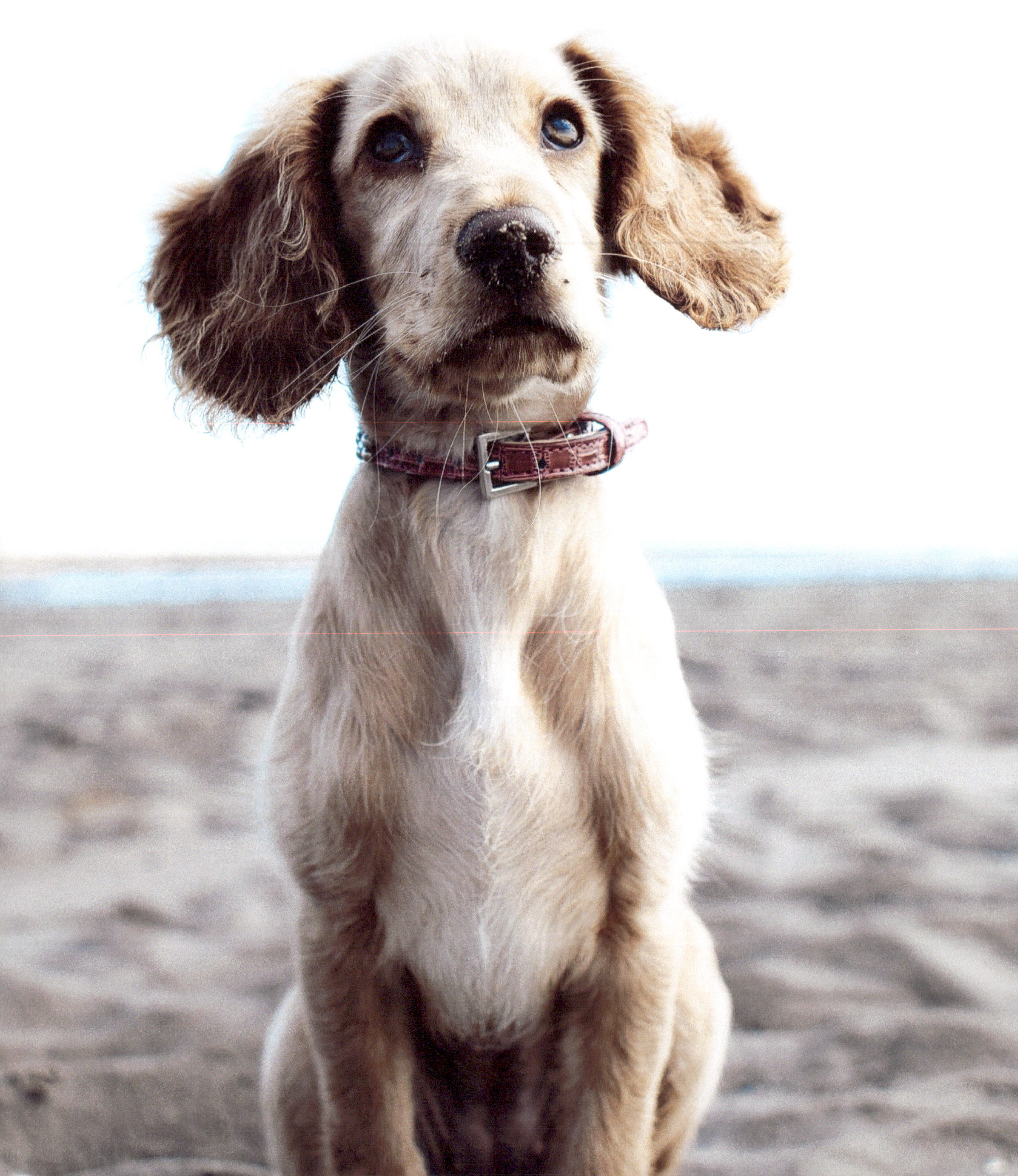

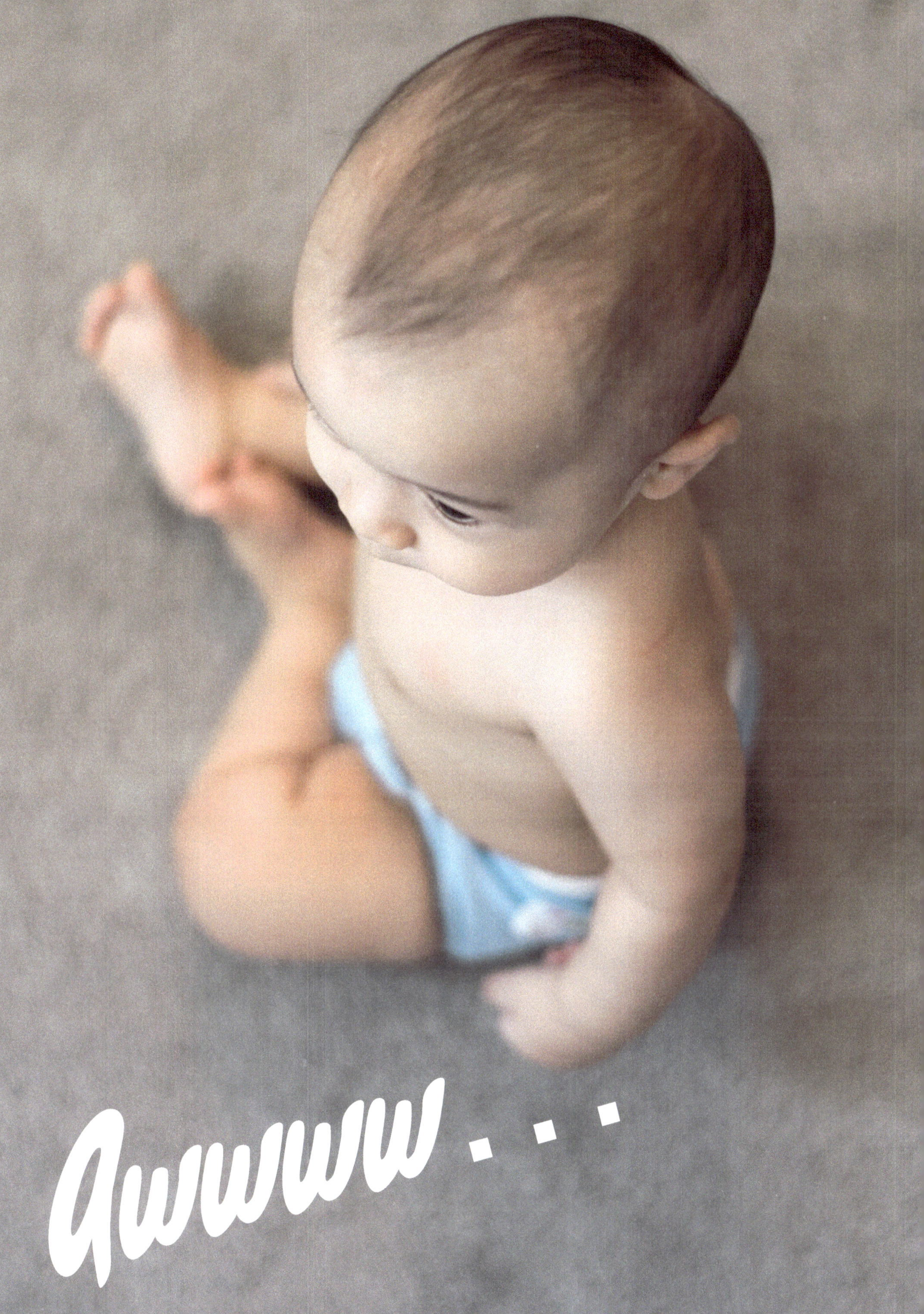
awwww . . .

Grounding Exercise
Sight plus Sound

Use videos like the following to your advantage. Make a quick link to playlists like these on your mobile phone or computer.

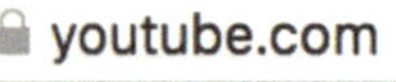

cute funny animals

About 10,100,000 results

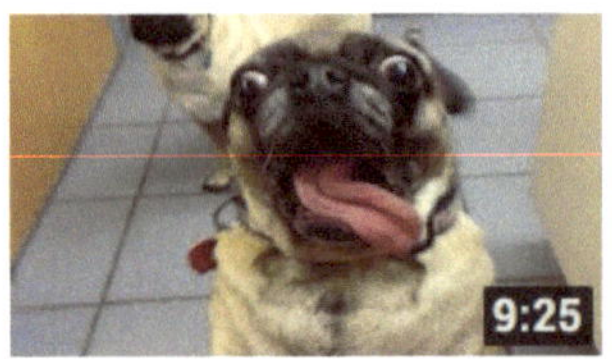

Animals are so funny that you can die of laughter - Funny animal compilation

Tiger Productions ✓ · 13M views · 1 year ago

Here is the best, **funniest**, **cutest** and most ridiculous **animal** / pet video clips collection. From **funny** cat fails, to monkeys, penguins,

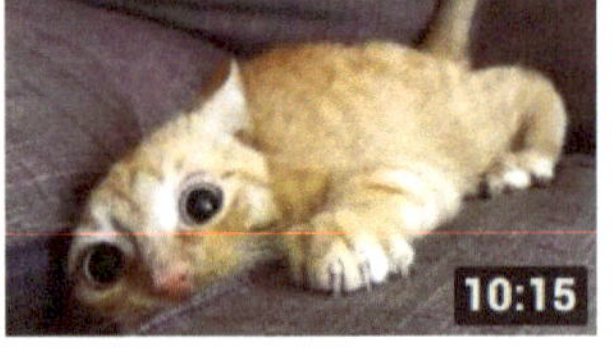

LAUGH UNSTOPPABLE at FUNNY ANIMALS - Super FUNNY ANIMAL videos

Tiger Productions ✓ · 620K views · 7 months ago

Only the best and the **funniest animal** videos! It's impossible to win this try not to laugh challenge! Just look how all these dogs,

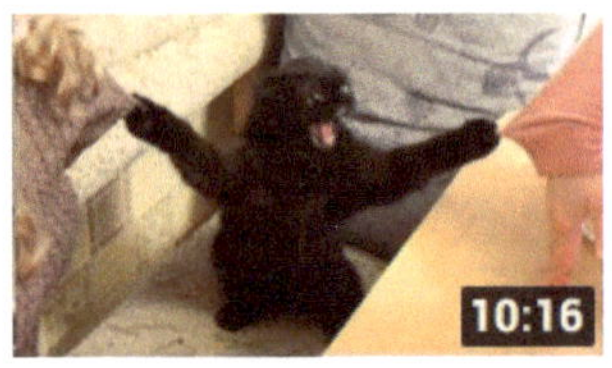

FUNNY ANIMALS: Try not to LAUGH - The FUNNIEST ANIMAL videos

Tiger Productions ✓ · 1.7M views · 4 months ago

Just look how all these dogs, puppies, cats, kittens, goats, horses,... behave, play, fail, make **funny** sounds, react to different things,...

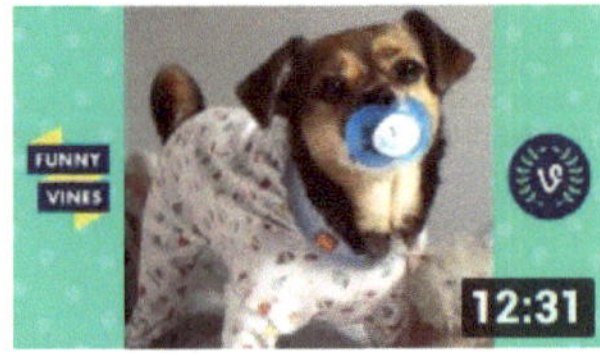

Funny Animals Vines V2 March 2018 Compilation | Cute Pets, Dogs, Birds, Cats Videos Monthly Montage

Funny Vines ✓ · 1.4M views · 1 month ago

Funny Vines of March 2018 **Animal** Edition! This fpv monthly compilation features **funny** pets including cats, dogs, puppies, kittens,

Grounding Exercise
Hearing

Listen to your surroundings.

What is one thing you can hear?

What is a second thing you can hear?

What do you like to hear?

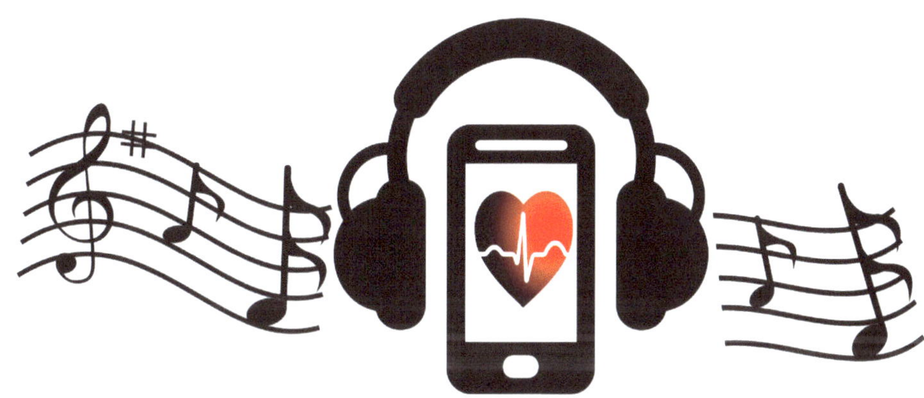

One choice might be music. A person's heart rate changes while listening to music, but the rate depends on the tempo of the music. An average resting heart rate is about 70 beats per minute. When you are anxious your heart rate is probably above a resting rate, so you may need to reduce it. **Find some mellow music to help you relax and lower your heart rate.** You can even find music online that is listed in playlists by beats per minute.

Brain Games
Mental Exercises

Count backward from 30 to 0

30, 29, 28, 27 …

Don't look down at your feet. **What shoes are you wearing?**
What color are they? Where did you get them?
Wiggle your toes. Try to move your toes one at a time.

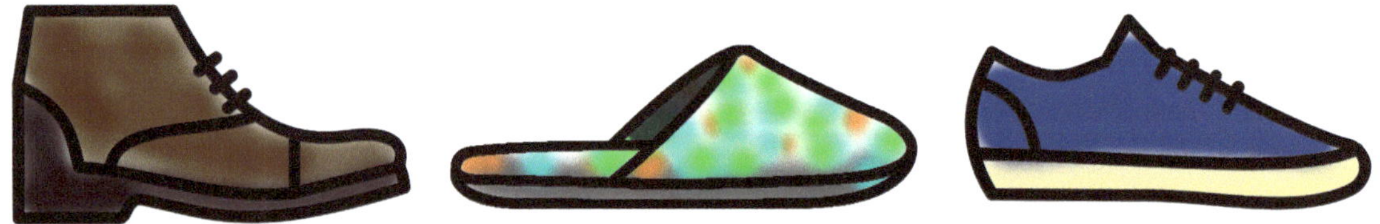

Don't look down! **What clothes are you wearing?**
How long have you owned them? Are they comfortable? Relax
your arms and legs one at a time. Walk around and notice how
your feet feel, how your shoes feel, how the texture of your
clothes feel. Too loose? Too tight? Springy? Smooth?

Brain Games
Imagery

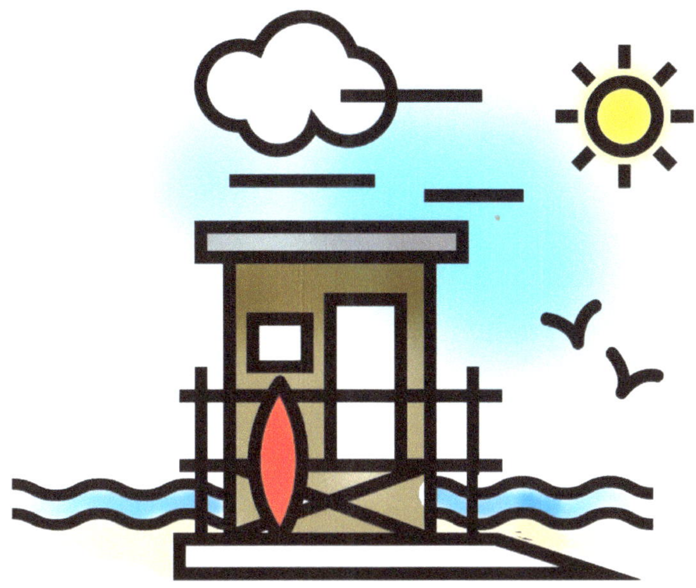

Get comfortable in a chair or lie down. Breathe deeply.
Begin to create a picture in your mind of a place where you like
to relax. Where is this peaceful place? Imagine details of your
surroundings. Focus on the relaxing sounds around you in your
peaceful place. Now imagine any tastes and smells. Is it cool or
warm and sunny? Breezy or still? What would you be doing in
this calming place? Imagine you are happy and peaceful.
Close your eyes for a few minutes, keeping this image in your
mind and breathing deeply and slowly.

This completes all your calming exercises. By now, you are
feeling better, so just relax and listen to more music or **return
to whatever it is you want to be doing right now!**

Additional Resources
Apps

There are many free apps available to help you calm panic attacks. Some choices are Breethe, PanicShield, Breathbox, Headspace, Be Okay, Dare, Calm, Breathing App, PureMind and 10% Happier, to name a few. Download several now for quick access when you need them.

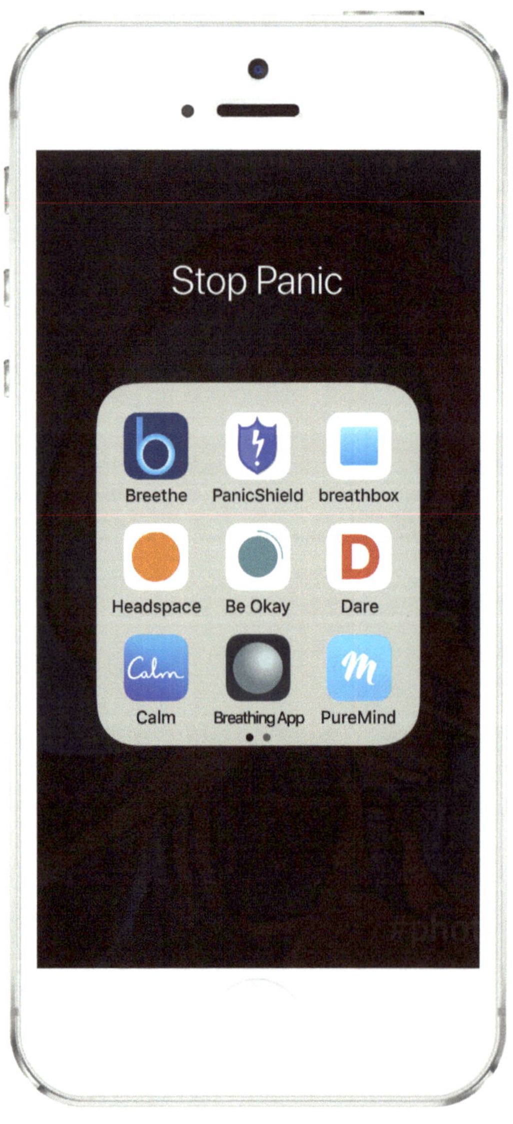

Additional Resources
Books

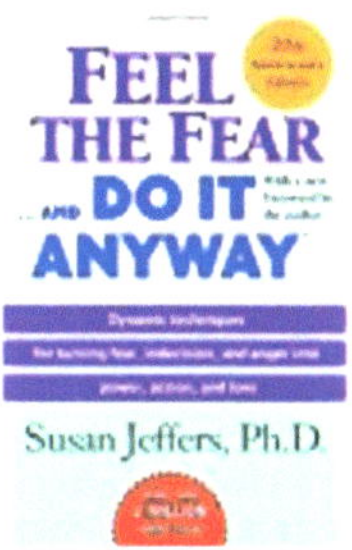

Feel the Fear . . . and Do It Anyway
by Susan Jeffers
★★★★⯨ ▾ (641)

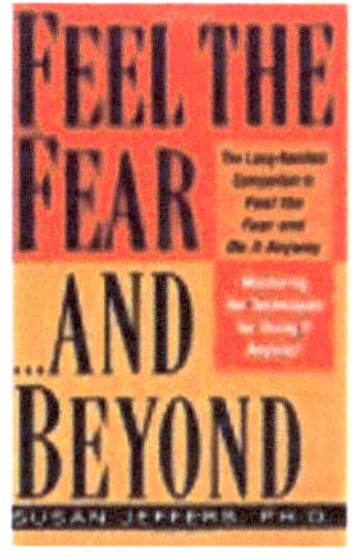

Feel the Fear.and Beyond: Mastering the Techniques for Doing It Anyway
by Susan Jeffers
★★★★⯨ ▾ (34)

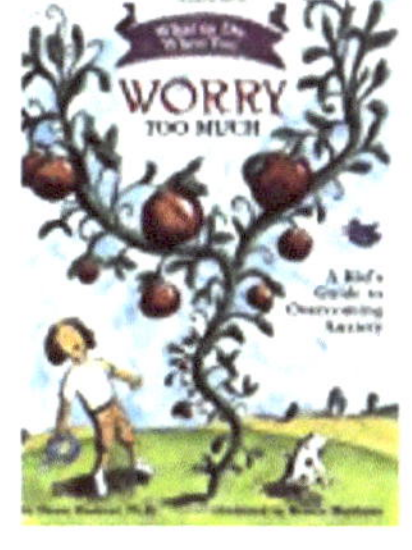

What to Do When You Worry Too Much: A Kid's Guide to Overcoming Anxiety (What to Do Guides for Kids)
by Dawn Huebner, Bonnie Matthews (Paperback)
★★★★⯨ ▾ (723)

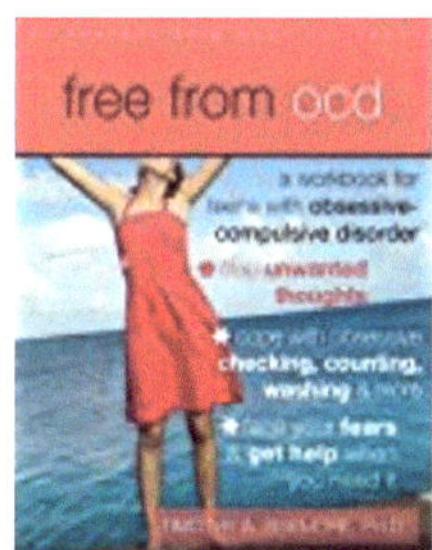

Free from OCD: A Workbook for Teens with Obsessive-Compulsive Disorder
by Timothy A. Sisemore
★★★★⯨ ▾ (19)

Did you enjoy this book?
Please consider leaving a review on Amazon.com.

This book is available in a video format.
Search for it on Youtube by typing
"Stop that Panic Attack Right Now, by Phyllis."